Carrier Oils

A beginner's guide to using over 40 carrier oils in bath and beauty recipes.

By Cari Dunn
Author of *Everything Pretty*
http://www.yourbeautyblog.com

Contents

What Are Carrier Oils? 1

Almond Oil.. 3

Apricot Kernel Oil 5

Argan Oil.. 6

Avocado Oil.. 7

Baobab Oil 8

Black Cumin Seed Oil 9

Borage Seed Oil... 10

Camellia Oil.. 11

Carrot Seed Oil... 12

Castor Oil 13

Corn Oil.. 14

Cranberry Seed Oil... 16

Coconut Oil 17

Evening Primrose Oil.. 18

Flax Seed Oil 19

Fractionated Coconut Oil 20

Grapeseed Oil 22

Hazelnut Oil 24

Hemp Seed Oil... 25

Jojoba Oil 27

Kukui Nut Oil.. 29

Macadamia Nut Oil 30

Marula Oil 31

Meadowfoam Oil 32

Moringa Oil 33

Neem Oil 34

Olive Oil 35

Palm Fruit Oil 37

Palm Kernel Oil 39

Passion Fruit Seed Oil 40

Peach Kernel Oil 41

Peanut Oil 42

Pecan Oil 44

Pomegranate Seed Oil 45

Pumpkin Seed Oil 46

Rosehip Seed Oil 47

Safflower Oil 48

Sea Buckthorn Oil 49

Sesame Seed Oil 51

Shea Nut Oil 52

Soybean Oil 53

Sunflower Oil 54

Tamanu Oil 55

Vitamin E Oil 57

Walnut Oil 58

Watermelon Seed Oil 59

Wheat Germ Oil.. 60

What Are Carrier Oils?

Carrier oils are vegetable oils made from the seed, nuts, or kernels of plants. They are so named because they carry essential oils and absolutes when they are applied to the skin. You may have heard them called base oils because they are the base upon which most bath and beauty recipes are created. Carrier oils are also used in sugar scrubs, lotions, balms, lip balms, soap, and salves.

You can't apply most essential oils directly to your skin, so you have to dilute them with a carrier oil. Using a carrier oil allows you to dilute essential oils in the right concentration for your application. Carrier oils also slow down the evaporation rate of essential oils so they last longer on your skin.

Carrier oils shouldn't have a strong smell, except for unrefined coconut oil. They will have a slight nutty aroma that doesn't usually affect your final product. If your oil has a strong odor, it could be rancid. Discard it and do not use it.

Carrier oils have different properties, so they each have unique benefits for your hair and skin. Some oils, like sweet almond oil and olive oil, are versatile and can be used in many recipes. Other oils, like avocado oil or neem oil, are used for specific reasons. If you substitute another oil, you won't get the full benefits of the recipe.

Shopping for carrier oils can be daunting, if only for the sheer amount of different oils available. This book will help you choose the right oil or oils for your recipes. It's not practical to own every oil there is, so use this book to help you select the carrier oils that will be beneficial for the most number of recipes.

When you're shopping for an oil, make sure you buy cold pressed oil if it is available. Heat can damage the good qualities of the oil, so it's very important to get cold pressed oils. Also look for unrefined oils with no additives.

The shelf life of carrier oils varies by the type of oil. Some have a short shelf life of only six months, and other are stable for a year or more. You should store your oils in an air-tight container out of direct light. Some oils need to be stored in the refrigerator after they are opened.

Carrier oils can go rancid. The amount of time it takes varies on the oil, the fatty acids, vitamin E content, how it was extracted, and how it was stored. You can identify a rancid oil by its smell. If your oil has a different odor, discard it and do not use it.

Keep in mind that your final recipe's shelf life will be dependent upon the shelf life of the products that you use. If you use an oil that is only good for 6 months and one that is good for a year, the product is only good for 6 months before it should be discarded.

Almond Oil

Almond oil is one of the most popular carrier oils. It's a mild hypoallergenic oil, so it is well tolerated by most people. It gets fully absorbed when you rub it on your skin, but it can still leave your skin oily for a few minutes after application.

There are two kinds of almond oil: Sweet almond oil and bitter almond oil, and they have very different functions. Sweet almond oil comes from the prunus dulcis, var. amygdalus tree, which is the same tree that produces the almonds that we eat. Bitter almond oil comes from the prunus dulcis, var. amara tree. Bitter almond oil is an essential oil and not a carrier oil, so do not use it in place of an oil in a bath and body recipe unless it specifically calls for bitter almond oil.

Almond oil is high in the essential fatty acids palmitic, palmitoleic, stearic, oleic, and linoleic acids. It is also high in vitamins A, E, and K.

Almond oil is a mild oil that is generally well tolerated by most people, so it's a good choice for sensitive skin. Since it's high in vitamin E, the oil can protect the skin against UV damage. The vitamin A can help prevent breakouts for those with acne prone skin. Almond oil is also a good oil to use on psoriasis and eczema because it has some anti-inflammatory properties.

The vitamins in the oil nourish the hair and the fatty acids moisturize hair, so it's a great hot oil treatment. It can also be mixed with other oils to be used on hair.

Apricot Kernel Oil

Apricot kernel oil is made from the seeds (kernels) of apricots. It's a light oil, so it's commonly used as a massage oil. It has a nutty aroma, but it's easily covered with essential oils. It's a versatile oil and works well in a variety of recipes.

Apricot kernel oil is high in vitamins A, C, and E. The oil is high in the essential fatty acids palmitic, palmitoleic, stearic, oleic, and linoleic acids.

Apricot kernel oil is an excellent moisturizer because it is an emollient, which means it helps keep the skin moisturized by preventing fluid loss. It is also said to have anti-inflammatory properties when applied to the skin. Apricot kernel oil is also said to be naturally antibacterial and a natural antiseptic. Apricot kernel oil is a gentle oil, so it's great for those with sensitive skin.

Since it's a lighter oil, it won't weigh down hair. It can be used alone or with other oils as a hot oil treatment to nourish and soften hair.

Argan Oil

Argan oil has been referred to as liquid gold because it is so beneficial for your hair and skin. Native to the Argan Forest in Morocco, this oil comes from pressing a nut from the argan tree to extract the precious oil.

Argan oil is high in vitamin E, vitamin A, fatty acids, and linoleic acid, which makes an excellent oil for both the hair and skin. These vitamins and fatty acids make it a wonderful tool for treating rashes, skin infections, and bug bites. When applied topically, the vitamin E in argan oil is said to boost cellular production while it nourishes your hair and skin.

Argan oil is one of the more expensive oils, but a little bit goes a long way. You'll only need a drop or two for your face or hair, and you can mix it with other oils for their benefits as well.

Avocado Oil

Most oils are pressed from seeds, but avocado oil is extracted from the flesh of the avocado fruit. Avocado oil can be used for cooking or applied topically to the skin. Avocado oil is rarely used alone in bath and beauty recipes. Instead, it's mixed with other oils, such as sweet almond oil.

Avocado oil is high in monounsaturated fats like oleic acid, vitamin A, vitamin E, vitamin E, and potassium. It also has antioxidants to help the body when ingested or applied to the skin. This oil is excellent for those with problem skin or sensitive skin.

Avocado oil is said to boost collagen production for firmer, smoother skin. This oil is unique in that it's one of the best oils to help the skin retain water, so it keep the skin supple, which can reduce fine lines. This also makes it a great addition to a lotion for dry skin. It's believed that the oil can help heal skin, so it's a good oil to use in an eczema cream.

Avocado oil is also a good oil for the hair and scalp. When massaged on to the scalp, it can stimulate hair growth while it nourishes hair.

Baobab Oil

Baobab oil comes from the seeds of the Adansonia tree in Africa. The trees are unique because they can live for 1,000s of years and look like they are growing upside down because the tops of the trees look like roots. The oil is cold pressed from the seeds and has been used for cooking oil in Africa for generations. However, it's best not to eat boabab oil unless it is specifically made for cooking because it can contain compounds that are toxic when ingested. Boabab oil is a thick oil with a mild smell. It feels silky on your skin, so it's used in cosmetics and as a moisturizer.

Boabab is high in vitamin A, vitamin E, and vitamin F. It has the saturated fatty acids palmitic acid, stearic acid, and arachidic acid. It's unsaturated fatty acids include oleic acid and linoleic acid.

It absorbs quickly into the skin, so it's a great oil for rough patches of skin. It is said to have anti-inflammatory properties and promote wound healing, so it's a good oil for dry skin. It's an emollient, so it helps moisturize skin while it promotes healing.

When used as a hot oil treatment, it leaves hair soft and silky. Many people notice more volume in their hair when they use baobab oil. It can also help protect hair from sun damage and prevent frizzy hair when used before spending time outside.

Black Cumin Seed Oil

Black cumin seed oil is also called black oil or black coriander oil. It comes from an Asian planted called the Nigella Sativa, which is part of the buttercup family and has black crescent shaped seeds. The oil is said to date back to the time of King Tut and Cleopatra, and Hippocrates was said to use it as well.

It's active compounds are crystalline nigellone, thymoquinone, palmitic acid, stearic acid, linoleic acid, myristic acid, oleic acid, arachidonic acid, and palmitoleic acid. It also has proteins, calcium, copper, zinc, phosphorous, folate, iron, and copper. It's also high in vitamins B1, B2, and B3.

Black cumin seed oil is said to have healing properties, so it's a good oil for eczema and scars. It also has antifungal and can combat yeast when used topically, making it a good oil to use in a foot cream.

Black cumin seed oil is said strengthen the hair follicle, which can help regrow hair for some people. It also makes a good hot oil treatment to soften hair.

Borage Seed Oil

Borage Seed Oil is a pale green oil derived from the starflower, a wildflower in the Boraginaceae family of plants. The Borage plant is an herb that is native to Syria, but it now grows in the Middle East, North Africa, Europe, and South America. Borage Seed Oil has been used for medicinal purposes for over 1,500 years. Borage Seed Oil blends well with essential oils and other oils, so it's a great addition to bath and beauty recipes. Heat can break down Borage Seed Oil, so don't use it in recipes that have to be heated. For best results, store in the fridge after opening.

Borage Seed Oil has protein, fats, vitamin A, vitamin C, riboflavin, choline, thiamine, and essential fatty acids. It's very high in gamma-linoleic acid, which is a polyunsaturated omega-5 fat that is excellent for your skin.

Borage seed oil is an excellent moisturizer and has some anti-aging effects on the skin. The fatty acids make it a good oil for eczema, dry skin, and psoriasis. It dissolves sebum, making it a good oil to use on the face.

Borage seed oil can also be applied to the hair to stimulate hair growth, but this hasn't been proven.

Camellia Oil

Camellia oil, also called tea seed oil, is made from the seeds of the Camellia sinensis, which is the plant that we get green tea from. Don't confuse this oil with tea tree oil, an essential oil from a different plant. Camellia oil is a light green color and has a sweet smell. Camellia has a long shelf life, but it should be stored in a cool, dark area.

Camellia is very similar to olive oil with its composition. Along with essential fatty acids, it also has vitamin E, phosphorus, potassium, and calcium.

Camellia Oil is an emollient, so it's a great skin moisturizer. It's also high in antioxidants, which is also great for your skin and can be a natural anti-aging product. It's also naturally antifungal and anti-microbial.

It is a great oil for skin irritations because it promotes skin healing and has a mild astringent effect on the skin. It's a natural pain reliever when applied topically, and it can reduce inflammation

Camellia Oil isn't often used in hair care because it is a heavy oil.

.

Carrot Seed Oil

Carrot seed oil was is made from the seeds of the carrot plant, native to India, France, and Egypt. The oil has a yellowish brown color and a light scent. Carrot seed oil is sometimes referred to as an essential oil, but I'm including it with the carrier oils because it's often mixed with other oils to create a bath oil or massage oil.

Carrot seed oil has camphene, a-pinene, b-pinene, mycerne, limonene and carotol. It also contains carotene, but it doesn't have vitamins A or E like carrots do as those are found in the root of the plant.

Carrot Seed Oil is said to help treat skin abscesses and boils. It can also tighten and rejuvenate skin.

Although I'm classifying Carrot Seed Oil as a carrier oil, it shouldn't be used alone on the skin. Always mix it with another carrier oil like olive oil or coconut oil. You should also do a patch test before using,

Castor Oil

Castor oil comes from the castor seed in India. The oil was used in Ancient Egypt, Africa, Greece, China, and Rome. In more recent times, it was used in the Americas and in Europe for it's many benefits.

The oil is fairly unique in it's composition because it is a triglyceride. It is high in fatty acids, and over 90 percent is ricinoleic acid. This fatty acid is also found in soybean oil and cottonseed oil, but it accounts for less than 0.3 percent of those oils.

Castor oil has many benefits for your skin because it is antibacterial, antifungal, and antiviral. When applied topically, castor oil, can help with dermatosis, acne, keratosis, warts, cysts, itching, and hair loss.

Castor oil is also said to boost your immune system when applied topically. Studies have suggested that castor oil can boost your lymphatic system, which can help rid your body of toxins and promote healing.

The fatty acids in castor oil are said to improve blood circulation in your scalp, which can help boost hair regrowth. It can also strengthen hair thanks to the nutrients in the oil.

Corn Oil

Corn oil is a common oil, and you'll find it in most every grocery store. The corn plant originated in Mexico and Central America, and it is grown all over the world now. Corn oil comes from the germ of the plant, which is the germinating part of the seed.

As with most oils, the cold pressed version of the oil is the healthiest and most expensive type of the oil. More often, corn oil is extracted from the germ by expeller pressing. The oil is treated with a solvent and then refined to remove the free fatty acids. Finally, it is steam distilled to get rid of some organic compounds. This process is more economical than cold pressing, but it can contaminate the oil with solvent and cause some of the healthy components of the oil to leave the oil. For this reason, it's best to use cold pressed corn oil and not the bottles that you buy from the grocery store.

Corn oil is high in linoleic acid, essential fatty acids, unsaturated fatty acids, vitamins E and K, and phytosterols, which are good for your scalp.

Corn oil is an emollient, so it is good for the skin. It makes a great massage oil when used alone or with other carrier oil or essential oils. Because it is high in linoleic acid, it penetrates the skin for more benefits. This makes it a great choice for lotions and lip balms.

The vitamin K in corn oil can help your hair, especially if

you have thinning hair. It also moisturizes dry hair and
tames frizzy hair.

Cranberry Seed Oil

Cranberry seed oil is cold pressed from the seed of the cranberry. Cranberry seed oil is often used in skin recipes for its many benefits.

Cranberry seed oil is high in vitamins A and E, essential fatty acids, phospholipids, phytosterols, and antioxidants. When used topically, it's said to help reduce fine lines and wrinkles and improve skin elasticity. It can also help prevent damage from the sun, but it should never be used as a substitute for wearing sunscreen. Because it is high in fatty acids, it's a great oil for dry, irritated, cracked, and itchy skin. It's often used in lotions for psoriasis and eczema.

Cranberry seed oil absorbs quickly into the skin and has a light fragrance. Because of the high concentration of vitamin E, it has a 2 year shelf life if stored in the fridge after opened.

Cranberry seed oil also has benefits for hair. It can strengthen hair and moisturize the scalp. It can strengthen hair and improve elasticity while it makes the hair shiny and smooths split ends.

Coconut Oil

Coconut oil is a popular carrier oil because of its wonderful smell. It's solid at room temperature, so it will harden a recipe when added. It can be heated and combined with other oils so the final product is softer.

When shopping for coconut oil, look for unrefined oil, which is the kind that smells like coconut. The refining process deodorizes and bleaches the oil, and it may also add sodium hydroxide to extend the life of the oil.

Coconut oil is high in medium chain triglycerides, a type of saturated fat. It is also high in lauric acid caprylic, and capric, three fatty acids that give coconut oil its antimicrobial properties. It is also high in the powerful antioxidant vitamin E.

Coconut oil is an excellent oil for your skin because it keeps it moisturized with the high concentrations of fats. It's antimicrobial properties make it a popular choice for salves and lotions, especially foot lotions. It's often used to heal dry skin

Your hair will also reap the benefits of coconut oil. Because of the fatty acids, coconut oil can penetrate the hair shaft to moisturize it. Use coconut oil alone or with other oils to tame frizzy hair while providing moisture.

Evening Primrose Oil

Evening primrose oil comes from the seed of the primrose plant. Primrose is a wildflower native to central and eastern North America. The seeds are cold pressed to produce evening primrose oil.

Evening primrose oil is high in essential fatty acids and gamma linolenic acid. It also has vitamin C for your skin. It is naturally anti-inflammatory, so it is a great oil to use on irritated skin.

Because of it's high fat content, evening primrose oil is an excellent oil for eczema and psoriasis. It's also said to help make the skin firmer and and reduce redness, so it's often used in facial recipes.

Evening primrose oil has been said to help hair regrowth when massaged on the scalp.

Flax Seed Oil

Flaxseed oil, sometimes called linseed oil, comes from the flaxseed plant. It's believed that the flaxseed plant has been harvested since 10,000 B.C., making this one of the oldest carrier oils It has a slightly sweet, nutty aroma that will blend well with other oils and ingredients in your recipes. Flaxseed oil should be stored in a dark bottle to prevent oxidation.

Flaxseed oil is 50 to 60 percent omega-3 fatty acid, specifically alpha-linolenic acid. It is also high in antioxidants.

Flaxseed oil is naturally anti-inflammatory, so it is a great oil for dry, irritated skin and psoriasis. It moisturizes the skin while keeping it hydrated. It's been said to help firm the skin and reduce puffiness. It can also help even skin tone, so it's a good oil for facial recipes.

Flaxseed oil can help promote hair growth and prevent hair from falling out. It is an excellent treatment for dandruff and flakes. Flaxseed also moisturizes your hair and makes your hair softer and look healthier.

Fractionated Coconut Oil

Fractionated coconut oil is so named because it is a fraction of coconut oil. Although coconut oil has a fairly long shelf life due to its saturated fatty acids, fractionated coconut oil has an even longer shelf life. Fractionated coconut oil is a liquid at room temperature, unlike coconut oil which is a solid at room temperature. The fractionated version of the oil doesn't have a scent, so it won't overpower other ingredients in your recipe.

To turn coconut oil in to fractionated coconut oil, most of the long chain triglycerides are removed, leaving the medium-chain triglycerides. This turns the oil into a saturated oil, which extends its shelf life and makes it more stable. This also increases the concentration of capric acid and caprylic acid to make it an excellent antioxidant with some antiseptic effects.

Fractionated coconut oil can not be substituted for coconut oil in most recipes because of the difference in consistency. It would be fine to switch them in sugar scrubs, but it might not give good results in soaps, lotions, or lip balms.

Fractionated coconut oil is an excellent skin moisturizer. It's often used for inflamed, irritated, or dry skin and for those with eczema or psoriasis. It can also be used in lip balms to heal chapped lips. It's generally tolerated by most skin types, including sensitive skin. Since it's nongreasy, it's a great oil for sugar scrubs and lotions because it will soak into the skin quickly.

Although fractionated coconut oil doesn't have a lot of benefits for your hair or skin, it's an excellent carrier oil because it mixes well with most other oils and essential oils. It's clear and odorless, so it won't overpower other oils. It's long shelf life means that your final products will last longer than if you'd used other oils.

Grapeseed Oil

Grapeseed oil is extracted from the tiny seeds of grapes, usually the same grapes that are used to make wine. Since it's a byproduct, it is a relatively inexpensive oil and can be found in most supermarkets. The oil is usually extracted chemically and not manually because grape seeds have a small amount of oil present in them. Grapeseed oil has a hint of nuttiness and is light in flavor and color. The oil should be stored in the fridge to extend its shelf life. It may congeal, but it is still safe to use until it smells bad.

Grapeseed oil is a polyunsaturated oil and contains linoleic acid, fatty acids Omega-3, Omega-6, and Omega-9, and vitamin E. It's high in oligomeric procyanidin, which is a powerful antioxidant. This antioxidant is stronger than most antioxidants, so grapeseed oil has a very long shelf life and can act as a natural preservative in beauty recipes. Note that it is not a strong enough preservative if you are using water in your recipe, so you should always use a preservative if you use water in your recipe.

Grapeseed oil has many benefits for your skin. It's a mild astringent, so it can help tighten pores and make large pores appear smaller. The antioxidants can help reduce sun damage and damage from free radicals. The oil is also said to help heal the skin due to the linoleic acid, which makes it a great oil for eczema and dermatitis.

Grapeseed oil is also an emollient, so it can help moisturize the skin.

For the hair, grapeseed oil can help make hair soft and smooth. It's also been said to promote hair growth when used on the scalp.

Hazelnut Oil

Hazelnut oil is made from cold pressed roasted hazelnuts. Hazelnuts are also called cobnut or filbert nut. The Hazel tree can be found in the Northern Hemisphere. The nuts grow in husks on the trees and fall out when they are ripe.

Hazelnut oil is high in oleic acid, linoleic acid, palmatic acid, stearic acid and also contains some linolenic acid. It is high in vitamin E, potassium, magnesium, and calcium. Because of its high concentration of vitamin E, it has a long shelf life.

Hazelnut oil is a great oil for acne-prone skin because it has antibacterial properties and is a natural astringent. It can help tighten pores while killing bacteria, so it's often used in anti-acne products. It moisturizes and condition skin to reduce the appearance of fine lines and wrinkles. Since it's a dry oil, it doesn't feel excessively oily on the skin.

Hazelnut oil offers some natural UV protection. It should never be used as a substitute for sunscreen when you will be in the sun and should only be used as sun protection in addition to your regular sunscreen.

This oil can help condition and strengthen your hair, so it's great for color treated or dry hair. It's often used it hair care to preserve color.

Hemp Seed Oil

Hemp seed oil comes from a the hemp plant. The hemp plant is the genus Cannabis, which is the same genus of plants that the drug is in. However, the industrial hemp plant that is used to make hemp seed oil is grown specifically for industry and does not contain THC, the substance that causes the psychoactive properties in the marijuana plant. This means that using the oil will not cause any drugs to seep through your skin and get into your system.

The entire hemp plant can be pressed for the oil, but the seeds produce the best oil. When cold pressed from the seeds, hemp seed oil is green and has a nutty flavor. After it is refined, the oil is colorless and has a faint odor.

Refining hemp seed oil strips it of some of its properties. It is often refined because unrefined oil does not have a long shelf life and can go rancid unless it is stored in the fridge. The refined oil is more shelf stable, so it can be purchased in larger quantities.

Hemp seed oil is comprised of polyunsaturated fatty acids. It also has vitamin E, carotene, calcium, sulfur, magnesium, phosphorus, zinc, and iron. It is also unique in that it contains chlorophyll.

The fatty acids in hemp seed oil moisturize and nourish the skin. It is often used for dry skin, eczema, acne, and psoriasis because of the fatty acids and minerals.

Hemp seed oil is also used in hair care. When used in shampoos and conditioners, it can thicken the hair and prevent dandruff. It can also help keep the scalp nourished to prevent flakes from dry scalp.

Jojoba Oil

Jojoba oil is actually a liquid wax and not an oil. It's a vegetable wax that is found in the jojoba plant, a tree that grows wild in the Southwestern region of the United States. Jojoba oil is colorless and odorless, so it's a great addition for many recipes. Jojoba oil is is a light golden color and has a slight nutty aroma when raw. After it is refined, it is odorless. Since it's a wax, it's not a greasy oil.

Jojoba oil is unique in that, unlike most other vegetable oils, it closely resembles sebum, a waxy substance produced by our skin glands. It can act as a natural skin conditioner, so it's an excellent oil to use in creams and lotions. It has nearly replaced animal fats in the manufacturing of skin lotions and creams because it is so close to the oil that we naturally produce on our skin.

Jojoba oil is a polyunsaturated wax. It's high in vitamin E, vitamin B, chromium, zinc, copper, and iodine. It also has the fatty acids oleic, gadoleic, and erucic.

Our skin secretes a waxy substance called sebum. When we don't produce enough sebum, we can get dry skin, dandruff, or itchy scalp. Jojoba oil mimics sebum in texture, so it can help relieve these conditions. Jojoba oil can also be used to remove excess sebum during puberty or due to hormonal changes. Jojoba oil is unique in that it can regulate sebum production for healthier skin, and it doesn't clog pores.

Jojoba oil is an emollient, so it moisturizes dry skin. It works by adding an oily layer on top of the skin to trap in moisture. Since it is high in iodine, it can also help destroy bacteria that leads to breakouts. The antioxidants in the oil can help fight signs of aging and reduce the look of fine lines.

Jojoba oil is a great oil for dandruff and dry scalp. It can also soften your hair and make your hair shiny when used in hair products.

Kukui Nut Oil

Kukui Nut Oil is cold pressed from the seeds of the Aleurities moluccans tree, which is also called the candlenut tree. It is the state tree of Hawaii, but it also grows in Polynesia. The oil can be almost clear to light yellow. Unlike most other oils, it should not be heated when used in recipes and should be added after heating other ingredients and letting them cool.

Kukui nut oil is comprised of linoleic and linolenic essential fatty acids. It is also high in Vitamins A, C, and E to nourish the skin and hair.

Since kukui nut oil is an emollient, it is an excellent oil for the skin, especially for damaged skin, psoriasis, and eczema. It doesn't leave a greasy film, so it makes a great addition to lotions or can be used on its own as a massage oil. When used in soap, it makes a creamy lather and makes the bar more conditioning. It's also been used to relieve the burn from radiation. The oil penetrates deep into the skin and creates a protective barrier on the skin, so it's excellent to use for windburned or sunburned skin.

Kukui nut oil can be used on damaged hair to nourish it and help restore it. It can also help restore hair that has been exposed to excessive sun and wind. Since the amino acids in the oil penetrate the hair shaft, it's a great oil to use on your hair as a leave-in treatment.

Macadamia Nut Oil

Macadamia nut oil is extracted from the macadamia nut. Macadamia nuts are a strong nut, and their oil retains some of their nutty flavor. It's amber in color, so it might change the color of your final product. It's a stable oil, so it has a longer shelf life.

Macadamia nut oil has one of the highest concentrations of palmitoleic fatty acid, which can help prevent the signs of aging. It also has oleic acid, linoleic acid, phytosterols, and sterols.

Macadamia nut oil contains squalene, which is an antioxidant that our bodies naturally product. Applying the oil topically can help slow the aging process, reduce wrinkles and fine lines, and prevent age spots. It also has anti-inflammatory properties, so it is a good oil to use after shaving or on irritated skin. This also makes it a great oil to use in lip balms.

This oil is also great for your hair and can make it look shinier and healthier. It can also strengthen the follicle in its bed, which can reduce hair loss.

Marula Oil

Marula oil comes from the nut inside the marula fruit. It's been used by women in Northern Namibia for skincare for centuries. It's a light oil that has a light texture and absorbs quickly into the skin. The pale yellow oil has an aroma that is both nutty and floral.

Marula oil has a high concentration of antioxidants, which makes it very stable. It has a high concentration of monounsaturated fatty acids, including oleic acid. Its polyunsaturated fatty acids are linoleic acid and alphalinolenic acid. It also has palmitic acid, steric acid, and arachidonic acid saturated fatty acids. It is high in vitamins E and C.

Marula oil is both anti-inflammatory and anti-microbial, so it's a great oil for damaged skin. It is also said to boost cellular turnover and reverse damage from the sun. It's not a greasy oil, so it's great for oily skin. It's also a good oil for sensitive skin. It's chemical composition makes it a great oil for stretch marks and scars.

It's an excellent oil for fine hair because it softens hair and reduces frizz without weighing down the hair.

Meadowfoam Oil

Meadowfoam oil comes from the meadowfoam plant native to Canada and the United States. The plant was considered ornamental until the 1950s when it was used for a renewable oil resource. It's a very stable vegetable oil and has a shelf life up to 4 years and can be refrigerated.

Meadowfoam oil is high in vitamin E, docosadienoic acid, and eicosenoic acid. It is similar to jojoba oil because it doesn't clog pores and balances oil on the skin.

Meadowfoam oil moisturizes the skin while forming a barrier on the skin to prevent moisture loss. It also has exfoliating properties, so it's an excellent oil for body scrubs. It's often used in anti-aging products because of its antioxidants and vitamin E, which can reduce sun damage. It also plumps the skin for more elastic skin to reduce fine lines and wrinkles as well as reduce scars and rough patches of skin. It's a non-greasy oil, so it's sometimes used as a massage oil.

The oil can help hydrate your hair and scalp while it makes hair look shinier and fuller. It can help reduce dandruff and flakes on the scalp.

Moringa Oil

Moringa oil is extracted by pressing the seeds of the Moringa oleifera tree, a tree native to the Himalayan area. This oil is also sometimes called ben oil because it is high in behenic acid. Moringa oil was used by the ancient Greeks and Romans, and it's still used today for its many skin and hair benefits.

Moringa oil is very high in antioxidants that help extend its shelf life. The oil will be stable up to 5 years, which is up to 4 years longer than most carrier oils. Moringa oil is also high in the saturated fats palmitic acid, stearic acid, arachidic acid, and behenic acid. It also has unsaturated fats oleic acid and some palmitoleic, linoleic, linolenic, and eicosenoic acids. Moringa oil is naturally anti-inflammatory when applied topically and a natural disinfectant. It absorbs the fragrance of essential oils, herbs, seeds, and nuts, so it's an excellent perfume base.

Moringa oil is often used in anti-aging products because it is so high in antioxidants. It is also used to heal skin because of it's anti-inflammatory and anti-microbial properties, so it can be used for eczema and psoriasis creams and lotions. These properties also make it an excellent oil for acne-prone skin because it can fight the bacteria that causes acne while reducing inflammation.

Moringa oil can also strengthen the hair by depositing vitamins and minerals to the hair shaft. This can make split ends appear better and tame frizzy hair.

Neem Oil

Neem oil is extracted from the fruit and seeds of the neem tree, an evergreen tree native to India. Neem oil has a bitter, almost antiseptic odor. The scent can be masked by using some essential oils though. Neem oil is often diluted with other carrier oils and not used on its own, usually in a 10 to 20 percent concentration of neem oil mixed with other oils. Neem oil can vary in color from yellow to dark brown to a bright red.

Neem oil contains the following essential fatty acids: linoleic acid, oleic acid, palmitic acid, stearic acid, alphalinolenic acid, and palmitoleic acid. It is also high in vitamin E and other antioxidants.

Neem oil is a natural astringent, so it's great for dry or itchy skin. It's also one of the best carrier oils for eczema, psoriasis, and acne because it moisturizes and reduces inflammation. Neem oil is absorbed into the skin quickly, so it's often used in beauty recipes. Neem oil is great for foot lotions and creams because it is naturally antifungal. .

For the hair, neem oil can help maintain a healthy scalp and healthy hair. When diluted with another oil, it can be used to massage the scalp to treat dandruff. It can also promote hair growth to combat thinning hair. The oil can also be used to condition hair and help with frizzy hair and split ends because it can temporarily close the hair cuticle.

Olive Oil

Olive oil is a popular carrier oil for beauty recipes because it is widely available in grocery stores. Olive oil comes from the olive fruit, which is native to the Mediterranean. There is evidence that people were making olive oil as early as 6,000 B.C. In the United States, extra virgin olive oil has the best flavor and odor and a concentration of 0.8 percent or lower of fatty acids. Virgin olive oil has a good taste and odor and a concentration of 2 percent fatty acids. If it is marked plain olive oil, it can be a mixture of virgin olive oil and refined oils. For this reason, you should buy your olive oil from a reputable source to ensure that it does not have refined oil in it.

Olive oil has oleic acid, linoleic acid, stearic acid, and palmitic fatty acids. It contains the powerful antioxidants vitamin E, polyphenols, and phytosterols, and it is also a good source of squalene, sterols, vitamins E and K, and iron.

It is a mild oil, so it is generally well tolerated by those with sensitive skin. Olive oil is a heavy, greasy oil, so it's not the best oil for scrubs or lotions because it takes a while to soak into the skin. Olive oil doesn't clog your pores, so it's an excellent oil for oil cleansing or for the face because it won't lead to acne.

Olive oil works well alone or with other oils as a hot oil treatment. It can help reduce frizzy hair and moisturize the hair, but it can be too heavy and make hair look oily or greasy.

Palm Fruit Oil

Palm fruit oil, also called palm oil, comes from the flesh of the palm fruit. The palm fruit is also where palm kernel oil comes from, but the oils have different properties. Palm oil has been used for 5,000 years due to its many benefits for the body. The oil is cultivated from trees found in both Africa and South America. Palm oil is naturally a shade of red. Colorless palm oil means that it has been stripped of its nutrients by processing it.

Palm fruit oil has been given a bad reputation because growers are clearing forest areas to grow the trees. This deforestation has displaced many animals, many of whom are becoming extinct. If you want to use palm oil in your recipes, please look for responsibly sourced oil.

Palm fruit oil is half saturated fat and 40 percent oleic acid, a monounsaturated fat. The rest of the fat is a polyunsaturated fat called linoleic acid. Palm fruit oil also has antioxidants, beta-carotene, and vitamins A, D, E, and K.

Palm oil's vitamin E comes from tocotrienols, which are stronger antioxidants. This makes the oil a great choice for anti-aging and fighting free radicals. The fats moisturize the skin and restore moisturize after washing, so it's often added to soap.

The vitamin E in palm oil promotes cell growth in the hair follicles, which can lead to stronger and thicker hair. The carotenes in the oil can also strengthen hair. The oils nourish the hair and make it soft, so it's also used in some hair products.

Palm Kernel Oil

Palm kernel oil comes from the same plant as the palm fruit oil, but it is extracted from the nutlike center of the fruit. Palm kernel oil is very similar to coconut oil in benefits, and and it is a semi-solid at room temperature. Just like with palm fruit oil, be sure to find a reputable source that does not destroy the natural forests to grow more palm trees.

Palm kernel oil is over 80 percent fat, mostly saturated fats. It also has lauric acid, which makes it have antimicrobial properties. It's high concentration of lauric acid also helps it lather, making it a great oil for soaps. It is also a good source of vitamins E and K.

Due to the high amount of vitamin E, palm kernel oil is often used in anti-aging products. It can protect your skin from sun damage and reduce free radical damage. It makes the skin soft without being too oily, so it's a popular choice for many beauty products.

Palm kernel oil can thicken hair and reduce hair loss by making hair stronger. It also helps nourish dry hair.

Passion Fruit Seed Oil

Passion fruit oil, also called Maracuja oil, is from the passion flower plant, a plant native to Africa and South America that now grows in Hawaii and Australia. The seeds of the fruit are pressed to produce the yellow oil.

Passion fruit seed oil is is high in essential fatty acids linoleic acid, oleic acid, stearic acid, palmitic acid, and alpha-linolenic acid to nourish skin and hair. It also has vitamin C, phosphorous, and calcium.

This oil is wonderful for the skin because it can reduce redness and irritation, repair skin, and improve lines and wrinkles. It can also help boost collagen production to improve skin elasticity and tone because of the vitamin C. The vitamin C can also help brighten skin.

Passion fruit seed oil can also be applied to the scalp to reduce flakes due to dandruff or dry skin. It can also be used to make dry, damaged hair look healthier when applied to the hair.

Peach Kernel Oil

Peach kernel oil is cold pressed from the pits of the peach tree. The peach tree is native to China, but it was brought to America by the Spaniards in the 1500s. It is similar to apricot oil in composition and application.

Peach kernel oil has polyunsaturated fatty acids, which are good for your skin when used topically. It is high in B-group vitamins and vitamins A and E.

Peach kernel oil is a light oil, so it's a good oil for the face. It can improve skin elasticity and reduce the signs of aging due to its vitamins. It absorbs quickly, so it can be used as a massage oil or combined with heavier oils.

Peach kernel oil doesn't weigh down hair and is easy to wash out, so it's a good oil to use on your hair. It coats the hair shaft to protect hair from the environment. It can also condition the hair to prevent breakage and reduce frizz.

Peanut Oil

Peanut oil is made from a low-growing plant called Arachis hypogea. The peanut is actually a legume that grows underground and not a nut like its name implies. It is believed that peanuts are native to South America and that the Incans used them. It now grows in North America, Africa, and Asia. Peanut oil has a deep yellow color and sweet, nutty fragrance when it is cold pressed. When it is refined, it is light yellow and has a neutral taste.

Although the part of the peanut that most people with a peanut allergy react to is not present in the oil, avoid peanut oil if you or anyone you will be around has a peanut allergy.

Peanut oil is high in unsaturated fats, the most prominent of which are oleic acid and linoleic acid. It also has some saturated fat. It has antioxidants in it, including vitamin E. It also has vitamins A and D.

Thanks to its vitamin E, peanut oil can be used to prevent the signs of aging, including fine lines and wrinkles. Peanut oil has some anti-inflammatory properties when used topically. It is unique in that it creates a barrier preventing air and water from moving through it, which is helpful for wounds. Peanut oil is an analgesic and can reduce pain when used topically.

When massaged on the scalp, peanut oil can help control flakes and psoriasis. Peanut oil may increase hair strength and reduce hair loss when massaged on the scalp. The protein in the oil can make hair healthier and shinier when applied to the hair.

Pecan Oil

Pecans are a tree nut native to North America. The Native Americans in the south and central parts of the country used pecan oil in several natural remedies. The oil is cold-pressed from the pecan kernel and has little to no odor.

Pecan oil is high in vitamins A and E, zinc, phosphorus, and folate. It's also high in antioxidants to help your skin. Pecan oil is high in essential fatty acids linoleic acid, oleic acid, palmitic acid, stearic acid, and linolenic acid.

The antioxidants in pecan oil fight free radicals, so it's a good oil for the skin. It can help reduce the appearance of fine lines and wrinkles. The vitamin A can help clear the complexion, and the zinc can keep skin healthy.

Pecan oil can stimulate hair growth when massaged on to the scalp. It can also strengthen hair and increase the density of hair when used for several months.

Pomegranate Seed Oil

Pomegranate seed oil comes from the seed of the fruit from the small tree Punica granatum. The seeds are pressed to extract the oil. The oil can also be extracted using heat, but this can destroy some of the nutritional benefit of the oil. The oil has a fruity fragrance and a soft amber color.

Pomegranate seed oil is high in antioxidants to combat free radicals. It can also stimulate the production of skin cells to promote healthier skin. It is high in the omega-5 fatty acid punicic acid, which can reduce inflammation from eczema, psoriasis, and acne. It is also high in vitamin C.

This oil is a great choice for an anti-aging oil because of the antioxidants. It can also help regulate sebum production, so it's often used for facial creams and serums. It has many healing properties, making it a good oil for sunburns, eczema, psoriasis, cuts, and cracked skin. It helps promote skin cell turnover and prevents the breakdown of collagen to combat the signs of aging. Vitamin C helps improve skin elasticity and skin tone.

The punicic acid in pomegranate oil helps strengthen hair. When massaged on the scalp, it can improve blood circulation to promote hair growth. It can help reduce itchy scalp and reduce dandruff.

Pumpkin Seed Oil

Pumpkin seed oil is made from several varieties of pumpkins, but it is usually made from the Cucurbita pepo var styriaca pumpkin plant. The oil can be cold pressed or obtained through a solvent. Cold pressed oil is healthier, but it has a lower yield, which raises the cost of the oil. Pumpkin seed oil can be dark green or deep red in color. Usually, the two colors mix to make a dark green or black oil.

Pumpkin seed oil is high in vitamins A, E, and K, iron, selenium, and zinc. It also has omega-6 fatty acids to improve hair and skin health.

Pumpkin oil can be applied directly to the skin or used in other recipes. The fatty acids and antioxidants soften the skin while promoting skin regeneration. It's been said to increase firmness and improve eczema. The zinc and selenium can help clear acne prone skin. Pumpkin seed oil has a great consistency to be used as a massage oil, and it can be combined with other oils.

It can also be used on the scalp and left on for up to 2 hours to soothe an irritated scalp. It's best not to use it on greasy scalps because it can be too heavy. It also helps improve hair health and makes hair shiny while it hydrates the hair follicle. It is a great oil to use on damaged or processed hair.

Rosehip Seed Oil

Rosehip seed oil comes from the rosehip fruit, a plant that is native to Chile. The oil was used by the Native Americans, Mayans, and even the Ancient Egyptians for its healing properties when used topically. As with most carrier oils, the cold pressed variety is superior because it doesn't lose its nutritional value.

Rosehip seed oil is high in essential fatty acids linoleic acid and linolenic acid and vitamins A and E. It also has antioxidants and vitamins A and C to improve the skin.

Because it has natural vitamins A and C, it can correct UV damage from the sun and even out skin tone. It also works well on fine lines and wrinkles to reduce the signs of aging. Many people love it to use on their faces, but it is also a good oil for psoriasis, eczema, scars, and dry skin. It is also a great oil to use on nails because it moisturizes and strengthens toenails and fingernails.

Rosehip oil absorbs quickly, so it's a good choice for a dry or flaky scalp. It's a light oil, so it's a good oil for a hair mask. It seals moisture into the hair without making it overly greasy or oily.

Safflower Oil

Safflower is a thistle-like plant that is not known to have any other uses than its oil. The plant was used by the Greeks and Egyptians for its seeds, which were used to dye fabrics. Today, the plant is only used for its oil.

Safflower oil is the highest source of polyunsaturated fats of any vegetable oil and has almost 80 percent linoleic acid. It also has the monounsaturated fat oleic acid and some saturated fatty acids. It also contains vitamins E and K and a small amount of choline.

Safflower oil is often used for oil cleansing because the linoleic acid combines with sebum to unclog the pores and reduce acne and blackheads. This acid also helps promote the growth of new skin cells, so it's often used to treat scars and blemishes. The light, non greasy oil is an excellent moisturizer and is absorbed quickly. It doesn't clog pores, so it's a good choice for those with sensitive skin.

The oleic acid is also great for the hair because it can increase circulation in the scalp, which stimulates hair growth and strengthens hair follicles. It can also make hair stronger and shinier when applied topically. The vitamin E can help combat dry, brittle hair, especially hair that has been damaged from heat styling or chemical processing.

Sea Buckthorn Oil

Sea buckthorn oil has been used in Asia and Europe for centuries. It's believed to be native to the Himalayas, but it was mentioned by the ancient Greeks and Chinese as well as in Tibetan texts. The sea buckthorn is a shrub that grows in Asia and Europe.

There are two kinds of sea buckthorn oil: oil from the seed and oil from the fruit. The fruit oil is dark red or orange, and the seed oil is pale yellow or orange. Both have a musky scent. Both kinds of oil can be used topically, but the berry oil has more topical benefits, so it will be the oil that is discussed in this book.

Sea buckthorn berry oil is high in carotenoids and antioxidants. It also has vitamins A, C, and E, betacarotene, and several antioxidants. It also has copper, iron, manganese, and selenium. The oil is high in monounsaturated fatty acids and palmitoleic acid and palmatic acid. The oil is also naturally anti-inflammatory and anti-viral.

Sea buckthorn berry oil is a great oil for healing skin, so it's often used for eczema and psoriasis. Since it is naturally anti-viral and an anti-inflammatory oil, it can help prevent infections and reduce inflammation.

Sea buckthorn oil is best used on the hair when mixed with other oils like grapeseed oil, coconut oil, or olive oil.

It's amino acids and vitamins can help repair damaged hair, so it's often used as a hair mask or hot oil treatment.

Sesame Seed Oil

Sesame seed oil is extracted from the seeds of sesame. The yellow oil has a nutty flavor and has been used topically for many years. In ancient India, sesame oil was very valuable. It is believed that sesame oil is one of the oldest extracted oils in history.

Sesame seed oil is high in linoleic acid, oleic acid, palmitic acid, and stearic acid. It also has vitamins B, D, E and K.

Although sesame seed oil is heavier than other massage oils, it's still a great massage oil because it is said to detox the body. The oil is doesn't leave the skin greasy because it is readily absorbed into the skin. Sesame seed oil is also used on wounded or inflamed skin, so it's a great oil to use on eczema or psoriasis. It's often used a facial cream because of its antioxidants and antibacterial properties.

Sesame seed oil is a great choice for your hair as well as your skin. It can help detox your hair and repair damaged hair. It can also dissolve oil soluble vitamins and minerals on your scalp and in your hair. It can also be used in small amounts to restore shine to hair.

Shea Nut OIl

Shea nut oil shouldn't be confused with shea butter, which is a thick nut butter. The shea nut is native to Africa and has been used for skin and hair for 1,000s of years. Shea nut oil is a byproduct of the process to make shea butter. During extraction, a small amount of oil is produced. Unlike shea butter, shea nut oil is a liquid at room temperature, which makes it better suited to some recipes. High heat can lessen the shelf life of the oil, so it's best added to a recipe after it has cooled. The oil can be thick and hard to work with, but it can be thinned by placing the container in warm water.

Shea nut oil is high in palmitic acid, stearic acid, oleic acid, and linoleic acid. It is also high in vitamin E.

Shea nut oil absorbs quickly into the skin. It can be used alone or with other oils as a skin moisturizer all over your body. It's antibacterial and antifungal properties make it a great oil for dry skin or eczema. It is often used as a cuticle oil for dry or brittle cuticles.

Like shea butter, shea nut oil is also an excellent natural product for hair. It's a natural conditioner that works to make hair soft. It can also strengthen hair and improve growth rate. It helps seal split ends to prevent breakage and helps hair look less frizzy. When used all over your hair as a hot oil treatment, it can help restore shine and brilliance to hair.

Soybean Oil

Soybean oil is extracted from soybean seeds and is commonly used as a cooking oil all over the world. It also has a lot of benefits for the hair and body, and using it helps support American farmers. Light can reduce its shelf life and make it go rancid, so be sure to store it in a dark bottle in a dark place.

Soybean oil is high in linoleic acid and linolenic acid. It's also high in B vitamins and vitamins A, C, E and K. Ferulic acid in soybean oil helps improve skin health. Soybean oil contains iron, zinc, selenium, phosphorus, magnesium, copper, calcium, and manganese.

When using soybean oil topically, look for organic oil because it is milder and is less likely to irritate skin. Soybean oil is often used topically because it can help reverse sun damage and help skin look healthy. The antioxidants help protect skin from free radicals and is usually included in anti-aging recipes.

Organic soybean oil can also be used on hair to make it stronger and shinier. It's often used alone or with other carrier oils as a hot oil treatment for stronger, softer hair.

Sunflower Oil

Sunflowers are native to America. The oil is extracted from the seeds and used for cosmetics and for cooking. The oil is amber in color, and the refined oil is pale yellow. It has a long shelf life, so it's a popular oil for recipes.

Sunflower oil is high in linoleic acid, oleic acid, stearic acid, and palmitic acid. It also contains vitamins A, B, C D, and E, lecithin, carotenoids, and tocopherols. Sunflower oil also contains waxes, lecithin, calcium, iron, and potassium.

Sunflower oil is an emollient, so it traps moisture against the skin. The vitamin E content in the oil makes it a good oil for anti-aging, and it can help reduce the signs of aging like fine lines and wrinkles. The linoleic acid helps decrease inflammation from acne, sunburns, and dermatitis. The oil is generally well tolerated, so it is a good oil to use under the eyes and on sensitive skin.

When used on hair, sunflower oil conditions and softens hair while making it shinier and more manageable. Since it's a light oil, it penetrates the hair shaft to nourish hair and repair damage.

Tamanu Oil

Tamanu oil is extracted from the nut kernels of the tamanu tree. The tamanu tree is native to Southeast Asia in Vietnam, Thailand, Sri Lanka, Malaysia, South India, and the Polynesian islands. After the tree grows an apple like fruit, the kernel of the fruit is sun dried for several months and then cold pressed to produce at yellow-green oil with a nutty fragrance. The oil is expensive because the trees are slow growing, and it takes many kernels to get a few ounces of oil. For this reason, the oil is often diluted with another carrier oil when used in recipes.

The oil is high in linoleic acid, oleic acid, stearic acid, and palmitic acid. It also contains vitamins A and E and several antioxidants.

Tamanu oil has enzymes that promote skin healing, so it's often used for skin conditions. It's a great choice to treat eczema, psoriasis, acne, and age spots. It can be used in a healing balm or stretch mark cream because of its fatty acids, vitamins, and enzymes. Its antioxidants make it a great oil for fine lines and wrinkles and to treat the signs of aging. The oil is thick, but it penetrates the skin quickly and doesn't leave a greasy residue.

The oil is also good for the hair and can be applied alone or with other oils to condition hair. It can seal split ends for better looking hair. Tamanu oil is a natural hair conditioner when used as a preshampoo oil or added to hair products.

Vitamin E Oil

Vitamin E oil, also known as tocopherol, is often combined with other oils to create beauty and skin care products. It is vitamin E in its purest form and is both an antioxidant and a nutrient that our skin and hair need. It's readily available at drugstores in capsules or liquid form. The capsules can be used in recipes by piercing them with a sterilized pin if liquid vitamin E oil isn't available.

Vitamin E is a nutrient that can benefit the hair and skin. It's an antioxidant, so it neutralizes free radicals.

The oil can be used alone on the skin to combat the signs of aging, including fine lines and wrinkles. It can boost collagen production and help skin cells regenerate quicker to reduce fine lines and wrinkles. It's also been said to help lighten brown spots on the skin and smooth rough skin.

VItamin E is often not used alone on hair but rather added to other products. It can be added to shampoo to soften hair and restore shine.

Walnut OIl

Walnut oil is extracted from English walnuts, and most of it is produced in California but it is made all over the world. The light colored oil has a nutty flavor and a delicate scent. It is a popular choice for massage oil and can be used alone, but it is sometimes mixed with other oils for their benefits.

Walnut oil is mainly made of polyunsaturated fats like alpha-linoleic acid, linoleic acid, and some oleic acid. It is high in antioxidants to fight free radicals in the body. It is a natural anti-inflammatory product, and it can also help kill bacteria and and fungus when applied topically.

Walnut oil can feel greasy when applied to the skin. It's a good oil to use on fine lines and wrinkles because of its fatty acids.

Walnut oil penetrates into the hair shaft, so it makes a good oil to use as a hot oil treatment. It can soften hair and make it more manageable, and the potassium can help cells regenerate to improve hair growth.

Watermelon Seed Oil

Watermelon seed oil comes from the Citrullus lanatus watermelon, which is the same melon that we eat in the summer. Watermelons are native to Africa, and the Africans are the ones who discovered the benefits of this oil. After the dried seeds are pressed, a yellow oil emerges. It is a light, stable oil with a nutty flavor that's often used as a massage oil or blended with heavier oils to make a recipe. It has a shelf life of a few years, so it's a great base oil to keep on hand.

Watermelon seed oil is high in palmitic acid, stearic acid, oleic acid, and linoleic acid. The oil is high in vitamins A and E as well as B vitamins. It also contains manganese, potassium, phosphorus, copper, iron, and magnesium.

Watermelon seed oil is light, so it's often used alone for massages. It is also used with thicker oils to bring them to a lighter consistency. The oil can dissolve sebum, so it's a good oil for oil cleansing or to be added to skin care products for acne-prone skin. It's often used for eczema and psoriasis because it's a gentle oil.

Watermelon seed oil can be applied to the scalp to reduce oiliness. When applied to oily hair, it can dissolve excess oil for better looking hair.

Wheat Germ Oil

Wheat germ oil is from the germ of the wheat kernel. The kernel is the center of the wheat berry, and it's what feeds the plant its nutrients. It has a strong aroma, so it's best used when blended no more than 10 percent with other oils. The oil should be stored in the fridge and has a one year shelf life. Wheat germ oil should not be used by those who are gluten-intolerant or allergic to wheat.

Wheat germ oil is high in vitamin E. In fact, it's one of the oil with the highest concentrations of vitamin E without fortifying the oil. It also contains vitamins A, B, D, and E. It's high in linoleic acid, palmitic acid, oleic acid, and linolenic acid. It's also a good source of protein, iron, and calcium.

Wheat germ oil is absorbed into the skin easily, so it's a good moisturizer. Because of its vitamin content, it moisturizes and heals skin. It's a good oil for very dry or cracked skin. The vitamins can also help prevent scarring. The high concentration of vitamin E can help support collagen production and fight free radicals, which can help defeat signs of aging.

Wheat germ oil can also help improve hair health. It's a good oil to use on frizzy hair and can help smooth split ends or broken hair. It's a natural emollient due to the long-chain fatty acids, so it helps add moisture to dry hair. The vitamins nourish hair while helping with hair growth for fuller hair.

For recipes using these oils, check out the DIY beauty recipes at Everything Pretty at http://www.yourbeautyblog.com.

www.ingramcontent.com/pod-product-compliance
Lightning Source LLC
Chambersburg PA
CBHW070846310526
45793CB00012B/673